Workout Journal For Women

Fitness Journal and Food Planner Diary in One

This Workout Journal Belongs To

_____

MY STARTING MEASUREMENTS

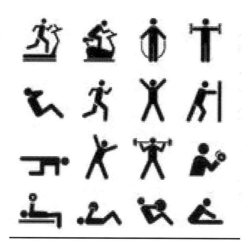

DATE	5/16/18
NECK	
BUTT	
WAIST	
HIPS	
BICEPS	
THIGHS	
CHEST	
ARMS	
WEIGHT	225

How To Use This Workout Journal

The journal is divided into two parts. On the right page, simply write the week beginning date at the top of the page and write everything down that you eat and drink on each day in that week. If you are counting your calories, you can write how many calories you consume each day too.

Summarize your week at the bottom of the page by writing about how you did overall. Anything that you want to write about your eating pattern, you put it in there.

The left page is for you to record your gym activity. Tracking your gym activity in this way is crucial as you will be able to see what you are doing and how this contributes to your overall fitness and health. It will become obvious what you need to do more of and also what is working well for you.

Write down the types of gym exercises and workouts that you do including the amount of sets and repetitions as you complete each one. In the notes section you can write a little bit about the impact of the individual exercises, your mood, your recovery after exercise, your water consumption, anything that you want to track.

Do not worry if you don't exercise every day, just fill this section out when you do with the date that you did the workout. (I bet you will not like to see this section blank and will exercise more just so you can fill it in). Summarize your week at the bottom of the page and track your fitness on a week by week basis.

This is your personal journal; it is a simple little diary for tracking a whole year's worth of workouts. By tracking your habits with this much detail you will become acutely aware of what you are eating and how serious you are taking your fitness goals.

This workout journal really gets under your skin and forces you to analyze yourself and make some positive changes in your life.

So what are you waiting for? Get started today!

WEEKLY WORKOUT / FITNESS JOURNAL

Date	Exercise / Activity	Sets	Reps	Notes / Summary
7/16	Airsquats	2	10	
	Plank Hold / Updowne		30 secs	
	Sit ups		10	
	Lunges		15	
	Step ups Onto Box		25	
	Goblet Squat		15	
	DB Thrusters pg 170	2	10	
	Jumping Jacks			
	Airsquats			
	Plank Hold / Up Downs			
	Mountain Climbers			
	Squat Jumps			
	Scissor Jump			

Summary of my week 1

Weight

Food Journal

DATE	Breakfast	Lunch	Dinner	Snacks	Total
Mon					
Calories					
Tue					
Calories					
Wed					
Calories					
Thu					
Calories					
Fri					
Calories					
Sat					
Calories					
Sun					
Calories					

Summary of my week

WEEKLY WORKOUT / FITNESS JOURNAL

Date	Exercise / Activity	Sets	Reps	Notes / Summary

Summary of my week

Weight

Food Journal

DATE	Breakfast	Lunch	Dinner	Snacks	Total
Mon					
Calories					
Tue					
Calories					
Wed					
Calories					
Thu					
Calories					
Fri					
Calories					
Sat					
Calories					
Sun					
Calories					

Summary of my week

WEEKLY WORKOUT / FITNESS JOURNAL

Date	Exercise / Activity	Sets	Reps	Notes / Summary

Summary of my week

Weight

Food Journal

DATE	Breakfast	Lunch	Dinner	Snacks	Total
Mon					
Calories					
Tue					
Calories					
Wed					
Calories					
Thu					
Calories					
Fri					
Calories					
Sat					
Calories					
Sun					
Calories					

Summary of my week

WEEKLY WORKOUT / FITNESS JOURNAL

Date	Exercise / Activity	Sets	Reps	Notes / Summary

Summary of my week

Weight

Food Journal

DATE	Breakfast	Lunch	Dinner	Snacks	Total
Mon					
Calories					
Tue					
Calories					
Wed					
Calories					
Thu					
Calories					
Fri					
Calories					
Sat					
Calories					
Sun					
Calories					

Summary of my week

WEEKLY WORKOUT / FITNESS JOURNAL

Date	Exercise / Activity	Sets	Reps	Notes / Summary

Summary of my week

Weight

Food Journal

DATE	Breakfast	Lunch	Dinner	Snacks	Total
Mon					
Calories					
Tue					
Calories					
Wed					
Calories					
Thu					
Calories					
Fri					
Calories					
Sat					
Calories					
Sun					
Calories					

Summary of my week

WEEKLY WORKOUT / FITNESS JOURNAL

Date	Exercise / Activity	Sets	Reps	Notes / Summary

Summary of my week

Weight

Food Journal

DATE	Breakfast	Lunch	Dinner	Snacks	Total
Mon					
Calories					
Tue					
Calories					
Wed					
Calories					
Thu					
Calories					
Fri					
Calories					
Sat					
Calories					
Sun					
Calories					

Summary of my week

WEEKLY WORKOUT / FITNESS JOURNAL

Date	Exercise / Activity	Sets	Reps	Notes / Summary

Summary of my week

Weight

Food Journal

DATE	Breakfast	Lunch	Dinner	Snacks	Total
Mon					
Calories					
Tue					
Calories					
Wed					
Calories					
Thu					
Calories					
Fri					
Calories					
Sat					
Calories					
Sun					
Calories					

Summary of my week

WEEKLY WORKOUT / FITNESS JOURNAL

Date	Exercise / Activity	Sets	Reps	Notes / Summary

Summary of my week

Weight

Food Journal

DATE	Breakfast	Lunch	Dinner	Snacks	Total
Mon					
Calories					
Tue					
Calories					
Wed					
Calories					
Thu					
Calories					
Fri					
Calories					
Sat					
Calories					
Sun					
Calories					

Summary of my week

WEEKLY WORKOUT / FITNESS JOURNAL

Date	Exercise / Activity	Sets	Reps	Notes / Summary

Summary of my week

Weight

Food Journal

DATE	Breakfast	Lunch	Dinner	Snacks	Total
Mon					
Calories					
Tue					
Calories					
Wed					
Calories					
Thu					
Calories					
Fri					
Calories					
Sat					
Calories					
Sun					
Calories					

Summary of my week

WEEKLY WORKOUT / FITNESS JOURNAL

Date	Exercise / Activity	Sets	Reps	Notes / Summary

Summary of my week

Weight

Food Journal

DATE	Breakfast	Lunch	Dinner	Snacks	Total
Mon					
Calories					
Tue					
Calories					
Wed					
Calories					
Thu					
Calories					
Fri					
Calories					
Sat					
Calories					
Sun					
Calories					

Summary of my week

WEEKLY WORKOUT / FITNESS JOURNAL

Date	Exercise / Activity	Sets	Reps	Notes / Summary

Summary of my week

Weight

Food Journal

DATE	Breakfast	Lunch	Dinner	Snacks	Total
Mon					
Calories					
Tue					
Calories					
Wed					
Calories					
Thu					
Calories					
Fri					
Calories					
Sat					
Calories					
Sun					
Calories					

Summary of my week

WEEKLY WORKOUT / FITNESS JOURNAL

Date	Exercise / Activity	Sets	Reps	Notes / Summary

Summary of my week

Weight

Food Journal

DATE	Breakfast	Lunch	Dinner	Snacks	Total
Mon					
Calories					
Tue					
Calories					
Wed					
Calories					
Thu					
Calories					
Fri					
Calories					
Sat					
Calories					
Sun					
Calories					

Summary of my week

WEEKLY WORKOUT / FITNESS JOURNAL

Date	Exercise / Activity	Sets	Reps	Notes / Summary

Summary of my week

Weight

Food Journal

DATE	Breakfast	Lunch	Dinner	Snacks	Total
Mon					
Calories					
Tue					
Calories					
Wed					
Calories					
Thu					
Calories					
Fri					
Calories					
Sat					
Calories					
Sun					
Calories					

Summary of my week

WEEKLY WORKOUT / FITNESS JOURNAL

Date	Exercise / Activity	Sets	Reps	Notes / Summary

Summary of my week

Weight

Food Journal

DATE	Breakfast	Lunch	Dinner	Snacks	Total
Mon					
Calories					
Tue					
Calories					
Wed					
Calories					
Thu					
Calories					
Fri					
Calories					
Sat					
Calories					
Sun					
Calories					

Summary of my week

WEEKLY WORKOUT / FITNESS JOURNAL

Date	Exercise / Activity	Sets	Reps	Notes / Summary

Summary of my week

Weight

Food Journal

DATE	Breakfast	Lunch	Dinner	Snacks	Total
Mon					
Calories					
Tue					
Calories					
Wed					
Calories					
Thu					
Calories					
Fri					
Calories					
Sat					
Calories					
Sun					
Calories					

Summary of my week

WEEKLY WORKOUT / FITNESS JOURNAL

Date	Exercise / Activity	Sets	Reps	Notes / Summary

Summary of my week

Weight

Food Journal

DATE	Breakfast	Lunch	Dinner	Snacks	Total
Mon					
Calories					
Tue					
Calories					
Wed					
Calories					
Thu					
Calories					
Fri					
Calories					
Sat					
Calories					
Sun					
Calories					

Summary of my week

WEEKLY WORKOUT / FITNESS JOURNAL

Date	Exercise / Activity	Sets	Reps	Notes / Summary

Summary of my week

Weight

Food Journal

DATE	Breakfast	Lunch	Dinner	Snacks	Total
Mon					
Calories					
Tue					
Calories					
Wed					
Calories					
Thu					
Calories					
Fri					
Calories					
Sat					
Calories					
Sun					
Calories					

Summary of my week

WEEKLY WORKOUT / FITNESS JOURNAL

Date	Exercise / Activity	Sets	Reps	Notes / Summary

Summary of my week

Weight

Food Journal

DATE	Breakfast	Lunch	Dinner	Snacks	Total
Mon					
Calories					
Tue					
Calories					
Wed					
Calories					
Thu					
Calories					
Fri					
Calories					
Sat					
Calories					
Sun					
Calories					

Summary of my week

WEEKLY WORKOUT / FITNESS JOURNAL

Date	Exercise / Activity	Sets	Reps	Notes / Summary

Summary of my week

Weight

Food Journal

DATE	Breakfast	Lunch	Dinner	Snacks	Total
Mon					
Calories					
Tue					
Calories					
Wed					
Calories					
Thu					
Calories					
Fri					
Calories					
Sat					
Calories					
Sun					
Calories					

Summary of my week

WEEKLY WORKOUT / FITNESS JOURNAL

Date	Exercise / Activity	Sets	Reps	Notes / Summary

Summary of my week

Weight

Food Journal

DATE	Breakfast	Lunch	Dinner	Snacks	Total
Mon					
Calories					
Tue					
Calories					
Wed					
Calories					
Thu					
Calories					
Fri					
Calories					
Sat					
Calories					
Sun					
Calories					

Summary of my week

WEEKLY WORKOUT / FITNESS JOURNAL

Date	Exercise / Activity	Sets	Reps	Notes / Summary

Summary of my week

Weight

Food Journal

DATE	Breakfast	Lunch	Dinner	Snacks	Total
Mon					
Calories					
Tue					
Calories					
Wed					
Calories					
Thu					
Calories					
Fri					
Calories					
Sat					
Calories					
Sun					
Calories					

Summary of my week

WEEKLY WORKOUT / FITNESS JOURNAL

Date	Exercise / Activity	Sets	Reps	Notes / Summary

Summary of my week

Weight

Food Journal

DATE	Breakfast	Lunch	Dinner	Snacks	Total
Mon					
Calories					
Tue					
Calories					
Wed					
Calories					
Thu					
Calories					
Fri					
Calories					
Sat					
Calories					
Sun					
Calories					

Summary of my week

WEEKLY WORKOUT / FITNESS JOURNAL

Date	Exercise / Activity	Sets	Reps	Notes / Summary

Summary of my week

Weight

Food Journal

DATE	Breakfast	Lunch	Dinner	Snacks	Total
Mon					
Calories					
Tue					
Calories					
Wed					
Calories					
Thu					
Calories					
Fri					
Calories					
Sat					
Calories					
Sun					
Calories					

Summary of my week

WEEKLY WORKOUT / FITNESS JOURNAL

Date	Exercise / Activity	Sets	Reps	Notes / Summary

Summary of my week

Weight

Food Journal

DATE	Breakfast	Lunch	Dinner	Snacks	Total
Mon					
Calories					
Tue					
Calories					
Wed					
Calories					
Thu					
Calories					
Fri					
Calories					
Sat					
Calories					
Sun					
Calories					

Summary of my week

WEEKLY WORKOUT / FITNESS JOURNAL

Date	Exercise / Activity	Sets	Reps	Notes / Summary

Summary of my week

Weight

Food Journal

DATE	Breakfast	Lunch	Dinner	Snacks	Total
Mon					
Calories					
Tue					
Calories					
Wed					
Calories					
Thu					
Calories					
Fri					
Calories					
Sat					
Calories					
Sun					
Calories					

Summary of my week

WEEKLY WORKOUT / FITNESS JOURNAL

Date	Exercise / Activity	Sets	Reps	Notes / Summary

Summary of my week

Weight

Food Journal

DATE	Breakfast	Lunch	Dinner	Snacks	Total
Mon					
Calories					
Tue					
Calories					
Wed					
Calories					
Thu					
Calories					
Fri					
Calories					
Sat					
Calories					
Sun					
Calories					

Summary of my week

WEEKLY WORKOUT / FITNESS JOURNAL

Date	Exercise / Activity	Sets	Reps	Notes / Summary

Summary of my week

Weight

Food Journal

DATE	Breakfast	Lunch	Dinner	Snacks	Total
Mon					
Calories					
Tue					
Calories					
Wed					
Calories					
Thu					
Calories					
Fri					
Calories					
Sat					
Calories					
Sun					
Calories					

Summary of my week

WEEKLY WORKOUT / FITNESS JOURNAL

Date	Exercise / Activity	Sets	Reps	Notes / Summary

Summary of my week

Weight

Food Journal

DATE	Breakfast	Lunch	Dinner	Snacks	Total
Mon					
Calories					
Tue					
Calories					
Wed					
Calories					
Thu					
Calories					
Fri					
Calories					
Sat					
Calories					
Sun					
Calories					

Summary of my week

WEEKLY WORKOUT / FITNESS JOURNAL

Date	Exercise / Activity	Sets	Reps	Notes / Summary

Summary of my week

Weight

Food Journal

DATE	Breakfast	Lunch	Dinner	Snacks	Total
Mon					
Calories					
Tue					
Calories					
Wed					
Calories					
Thu					
Calories					
Fri					
Calories					
Sat					
Calories					
Sun					
Calories					

Summary of my week

WEEKLY WORKOUT / FITNESS JOURNAL

Date	Exercise / Activity	Sets	Reps	Notes / Summary

Summary of my week

Weight

Food Journal

DATE	Breakfast	Lunch	Dinner	Snacks	Total
Mon					
Calories					
Tue					
Calories					
Wed					
Calories					
Thu					
Calories					
Fri					
Calories					
Sat					
Calories					
Sun					
Calories					

Summary of my week

WEEKLY WORKOUT / FITNESS JOURNAL

Date	Exercise / Activity	Sets	Reps	Notes / Summary

Summary of my week

Weight

Food Journal

DATE	Breakfast	Lunch	Dinner	Snacks	Total
Mon					
Calories					
Tue					
Calories					
Wed					
Calories					
Thu					
Calories					
Fri					
Calories					
Sat					
Calories					
Sun					
Calories					

Summary of my week

WEEKLY WORKOUT / FITNESS JOURNAL

Date	Exercise / Activity	Sets	Reps	Notes / Summary

Summary of my week

Weight

Food Journal

DATE	Breakfast	Lunch	Dinner	Snacks	Total
Mon					
Calories					
Tue					
Calories					
Wed					
Calories					
Thu					
Calories					
Fri					
Calories					
Sat					
Calories					
Sun					
Calories					

Summary of my week

WEEKLY WORKOUT / FITNESS JOURNAL

Date	Exercise / Activity	Sets	Reps	Notes / Summary

Summary of my week

Weight

Food Journal

DATE	Breakfast	Lunch	Dinner	Snacks	Total
Mon					
Calories					
Tue					
Calories					
Wed					
Calories					
Thu					
Calories					
Fri					
Calories					
Sat					
Calories					
Sun					
Calories					

Summary of my week

WEEKLY WORKOUT / FITNESS JOURNAL

Date	Exercise / Activity	Sets	Reps	Notes / Summary

Summary of my week

Weight

Food Journal

DATE	Breakfast	Lunch	Dinner	Snacks	Total
Mon					
Calories					
Tue					
Calories					
Wed					
Calories					
Thu					
Calories					
Fri					
Calories					
Sat					
Calories					
Sun					
Calories					

Summary of my week

WEEKLY WORKOUT / FITNESS JOURNAL

Date	Exercise / Activity	Sets	Reps	Notes / Summary

Summary of my week

Weight

Food Journal

DATE	Breakfast	Lunch	Dinner	Snacks	Total
Mon					
Calories					
Tue					
Calories					
Wed					
Calories					
Thu					
Calories					
Fri					
Calories					
Sat					
Calories					
Sun					
Calories					

Summary of my week

WEEKLY WORKOUT / FITNESS JOURNAL

Date	Exercise / Activity	Sets	Reps	Notes / Summary

Summary of my week

Weight

Food Journal

DATE	Breakfast	Lunch	Dinner	Snacks	Total
Mon					
Calories					
Tue					
Calories					
Wed					
Calories					
Thu					
Calories					
Fri					
Calories					
Sat					
Calories					
Sun					
Calories					

Summary of my week

WEEKLY WORKOUT / FITNESS JOURNAL

Date	Exercise / Activity	Sets	Reps	Notes / Summary

Summary of my week

Weight

Food Journal

DATE	Breakfast	Lunch	Dinner	Snacks	Total
Mon					
Calories					
Tue					
Calories					
Wed					
Calories					
Thu					
Calories					
Fri					
Calories					
Sat					
Calories					
Sun					
Calories					

Summary of my week

WEEKLY WORKOUT / FITNESS JOURNAL

Date	Exercise / Activity	Sets	Reps	Notes / Summary

Summary of my week

Weight

Food Journal

DATE	Breakfast	Lunch	Dinner	Snacks	Total
Mon					
Calories					
Tue					
Calories					
Wed					
Calories					
Thu					
Calories					
Fri					
Calories					
Sat					
Calories					
Sun					
Calories					

Summary of my week

WEEKLY WORKOUT / FITNESS JOURNAL

Date	Exercise / Activity	Sets	Reps	Notes / Summary

Summary of my week

Weight

Food Journal

DATE	Breakfast	Lunch	Dinner	Snacks	Total
Mon					
Calories					
Tue					
Calories					
Wed					
Calories					
Thu					
Calories					
Fri					
Calories					
Sat					
Calories					
Sun					
Calories					

Summary of my week

WEEKLY WORKOUT / FITNESS JOURNAL

Date	Exercise / Activity	Sets	Reps	Notes / Summary

Summary of my week

Weight

Food Journal

DATE	Breakfast	Lunch	Dinner	Snacks	Total
Mon					
Calories					
Tue					
Calories					
Wed					
Calories					
Thu					
Calories					
Fri					
Calories					
Sat					
Calories					
Sun					
Calories					

Summary of my week

WEEKLY WORKOUT / FITNESS JOURNAL

Date	Exercise / Activity	Sets	Reps	Notes / Summary

Summary of my week

Weight

Food Journal

DATE	Breakfast	Lunch	Dinner	Snacks	Total
Mon					
Calories					
Tue					
Calories					
Wed					
Calories					
Thu					
Calories					
Fri					
Calories					
Sat					
Calories					
Sun					
Calories					

Summary of my week

WEEKLY WORKOUT / FITNESS JOURNAL

Date	Exercise / Activity	Sets	Reps	Notes / Summary

Summary of my week

Weight

Food Journal

DATE	Breakfast	Lunch	Dinner	Snacks	Total
Mon					
Calories					
Tue					
Calories					
Wed					
Calories					
Thu					
Calories					
Fri					
Calories					
Sat					
Calories					
Sun					
Calories					

Summary of my week

WEEKLY WORKOUT / FITNESS JOURNAL

Date	Exercise / Activity	Sets	Reps	Notes / Summary

Summary of my week

Weight

Food Journal

DATE	Breakfast	Lunch	Dinner	Snacks	Total
Mon					
Calories					
Tue					
Calories					
Wed					
Calories					
Thu					
Calories					
Fri					
Calories					
Sat					
Calories					
Sun					
Calories					

Summary of my week

WEEKLY WORKOUT / FITNESS JOURNAL

Date	Exercise / Activity	Sets	Reps	Notes / Summary

Summary of my week

Weight

Food Journal

DATE	Breakfast	Lunch	Dinner	Snacks	Total
Mon					
Calories					
Tue					
Calories					
Wed					
Calories					
Thu					
Calories					
Fri					
Calories					
Sat					
Calories					
Sun					
Calories					

Summary of my week

WEEKLY WORKOUT / FITNESS JOURNAL

Date	Exercise / Activity	Sets	Reps	Notes / Summary

Summary of my week

Weight

Food Journal

DATE	Breakfast	Lunch	Dinner	Snacks	Total
Mon					
Calories					
Tue					
Calories					
Wed					
Calories					
Thu					
Calories					
Fri					
Calories					
Sat					
Calories					
Sun					
Calories					

Summary of my week

WEEKLY WORKOUT / FITNESS JOURNAL

Date	Exercise / Activity	Sets	Reps	Notes / Summary

Summary of my week

Weight

Food Journal

DATE	Breakfast	Lunch	Dinner	Snacks	Total
Mon					
Calories					
Tue					
Calories					
Wed					
Calories					
Thu					
Calories					
Fri					
Calories					
Sat					
Calories					
Sun					
Calories					

Summary of my week

WEEKLY WORKOUT / FITNESS JOURNAL

Date	Exercise / Activity	Sets	Reps	Notes / Summary

Summary of my week

Weight

Food Journal

DATE	Breakfast	Lunch	Dinner	Snacks	Total
Mon					
Calories					
Tue					
Calories					
Wed					
Calories					
Thu					
Calories					
Fri					
Calories					
Sat					
Calories					
Sun					
Calories					

Summary of my week

WEEKLY WORKOUT / FITNESS JOURNAL

Date	Exercise / Activity	Sets	Reps	Notes / Summary

Summary of my week

Weight

Food Journal

DATE	Breakfast	Lunch	Dinner	Snacks	Total
Mon					
Calories					
Tue					
Calories					
Wed					
Calories					
Thu					
Calories					
Fri					
Calories					
Sat					
Calories					
Sun					
Calories					

Summary of my week

WEEKLY WORKOUT / FITNESS JOURNAL

Date	Exercise / Activity	Sets	Reps	Notes / Summary

Summary of my week

Weight

Food Journal

DATE	Breakfast	Lunch	Dinner	Snacks	Total
Mon					
Calories					
Tue					
Calories					
Wed					
Calories					
Thu					
Calories					
Fri					
Calories					
Sat					
Calories					
Sun					
Calories					

Summary of my week

WEEKLY WORKOUT / FITNESS JOURNAL

Date	Exercise / Activity	Sets	Reps	Notes / Summary

Summary of my week

Weight

Food Journal

DATE	Breakfast	Lunch	Dinner	Snacks	Total
Mon					
Calories					
Tue					
Calories					
Wed					
Calories					
Thu					
Calories					
Fri					
Calories					
Sat					
Calories					
Sun					
Calories					

Summary of my week

WEEKLY WORKOUT / FITNESS JOURNAL

Date	Exercise / Activity	Sets	Reps	Notes / Summary

Summary of my week

Weight

Food Journal

DATE	Breakfast	Lunch	Dinner	Snacks	Total
Mon					
Calories					
Tue					
Calories					
Wed					
Calories					
Thu					
Calories					
Fri					
Calories					
Sat					
Calories					
Sun					
Calories					

Summary of my week

WEEKLY WORKOUT / FITNESS JOURNAL

Date	Exercise / Activity	Sets	Reps	Notes / Summary

Summary of my week

Weight

Food Journal

DATE	Breakfast	Lunch	Dinner	Snacks	Total
Mon					
Calories					
Tue					
Calories					
Wed					
Calories					
Thu					
Calories					
Fri					
Calories					
Sat					
Calories					
Sun					
Calories					

Summary of my week

Need another gym diary?
Visit www.blankboksnjournals.com

Made in the USA
Middletown, DE
26 March 2018